What I Have Learned From Coaching

What I Have Learned From Coaching

Timeless Prerequisites for Success and Fulfillment

Dennis Pursley

Library of Congress Control Number:		2022914495
ISBN:	Hardcover	978-1-6698-4172-2
	Softcover	978-1-6698-4171-5
	eBook	978-1-6698-4170-8

Cover photo:
1980 U.S. Olympic Trials
100 meter butterfly awards presentation
Mary T. Meager, Tracy Caulkins, Ronald Reagan, Lisa Buese

Print information available on the last page.

Rev. date: 09/28/2022

To order additional copies of this book, contact:
Xlibris
844-714-8691
www.Xlibris.com
Orders@Xlibris.com
845019

Contents

PART III: PERFORMANCE EXCELLENCE

PART IV: SUCCESS AND FULFILLMENT

Regardless of the outcome, it is through the process of striving
to achieve our worthy goals and to become better people
that we experience personal growth.
When we stop striving, we stop growing.

Introduction

As a competitive swimmer, I was very fortunate to have been coached and mentored at the Plantation Swim Club in Louisville, Kentucky, by a man of the highest integrity, Ralph Wright. Coach Wright instilled in his swimmers many of the attributes that I will be referring to in this book. Together with that of my parents, his influence has had an immeasurable impact on any success I have had in my professional career.

During my fifty-year coaching tenure, I was privileged to have had the opportunity to work with a full spectrum of athletes, teams, and colleagues, ranging from novice swimmers and rookie coaches to some of the most accomplished athletes, coaches, and teams in the history of our sport. Each of these experiences was unique and special in its own way, and each taught me valuable life lessons.

While serving a one-year apprenticeship as a volunteer coach under Coach Don Gambril at my alma mater, the University of Alabama, I spent all my free time absorbing the wisdom of the masters in our profession through the books they had written and transcripts of the presentations they had given at various coaches' clinics. Coach Gambril was one of these coaches and he was a no-nonsense coach. The team goals and expectations were clearly articulated, as were the consequences for failing to live up to those expectations. More importantly, those consequences were enforced. We quickly learned that we would be held accountable to do our part.

The process of searching for my first post-graduate professional coaching opportunity taught me that sometimes, our greatest disappointments in life can actually be blessings in disguise. I thought I was well prepared for my interviews but failed to secure a job offer for any of the positions that I had applied for. Just as I was at the point of despair and questioning whether I should abandon my intention to pursue a coaching career, I was offered a head coaching position at Lakeside Swim Club in Louisville. At that time, Lakeside was starting a rebuilding phase in its program history, but it had unlimited potential. None of the positions that I had previously applied for had nearly the same level of potential. Had I been offered any of them, I would have accepted the offer and my career path would likely have been very different. Again, a blessing in disguise. I have since advised young coaches to consider potential and opportunity above all else (salary, location, current ranking, etc.) in making career choices. By fully developing the potential of a program, these other benefits and rewards will follow. The greater the potential, the greater the rewards.

When I was offered my first head coaching position, I reached out to four of the most accomplished coaches in our sport and asked them what I needed to do to be successful in my career. To my surprise, they all said that I needed to surround myself with loyal, committed, and enthusiastic assistant coaches. Years of experience have taught me the significance of this advice. No team effort has a chance of succeeding unless all team members, beginning with the leaders, are on the same page and supporting one another in the pursuit of the team goals. I had to put this advice on hold, however, because I had no assistants when I first started at Lakeside. I was a one-man show. As challenging as that was, it was an invaluable learning experience for me as I was directly responsible for all aspects of the program. Baptism by fire!

The first lesson I learned as a rookie head coach was the importance of holding the swimmers accountable to comply with expectations. I was working with a group of enthusiastic young athletes who were excited about our new beginning but had developed sloppy training habits. Taking a page from my mentor, Coach Gambril, I clearly articulated the training expectations. I talked repeatedly about these expectations, but my instructions went in one ear and out the other. Realizing that our performance goals would not be achieved unless this problem was resolved, I informed them that, moving forward, noncompliance would result in indefinite suspension from the team. Old habits die hard, so most of the swimmers in the group were suspended in short order. I was worried that my coaching career was already in jeopardy but was relieved to discover that all the suspended swimmers accepted my invitation to meet with me one-on-one to discuss the terms and conditions required to be reinstated in the group. The message was received, and I was soon coaching a team in a much more focused and professional training environment. Lack of accountability will lead to a failure to adapt and adjust, a failure to respect authority, and a failure to step up to a challenge and respond effectively to adversity.

Knowing that performance results are sometimes dependent on factors and circumstances that we can't always control, I decided to put the emphasis on effort over performance results, believing that the results would eventually follow if the effort was consistent, both in practice and in competition. We adopted Winston Churchill's mantra as our team mandate: "Never, never, never quit." The team embraced this mindset with pride and determination. It contributed significantly to our progress, both as individual athletes and as a team. Although we established performance goals for our team and our athletes, success and failure were not defined by those arbitrary goals. They were used as incentives to inspire our swimmers to strive to be the best that they could be. This was the ultimate goal by which success was measured, and it was attainable by ALL the swimmers regardless of their level of talent and ability. By this measure, I have observed Olympic champions who were not as successful as some lower-level athletes who came closer to achieving their full potential.

My coaching experience with this team also taught me the value of enthusiasm. I was familiar with training physiology and performance standards for collegiate males but was not familiar with performance standards for age group or high school swimmers. This turned out to be another blessing in disguise. Since I was not yet familiar with national or regional level standards for these swimmers, I used their previous best performances as the standards by which to evaluate their performances. Each time they achieved a personal best, I reacted as if they had broken a world record. (In fact, I probably reacted with less enthusiasm in later years when my swimmers DID break world records.) The swimmers responded by redoubling their efforts to achieve a personal best at the next opportunity to elicit the same reaction. Had I realized what a low bar of achievement I was responding to, my enthusiasm would likely have been substantially diminished and so would the response of the swimmers. As it was, we fed off one another's enthusiasm, and it wasn't long before they were performing at the regional and national level.

In year three of our rebuilding plan, I believed that our fastest swimmers were finally within reach of achieving the qualifying standards required to compete in the national championships. We traveled with high expectations to Bloomington, Indiana, to compete in a national championship qualifying meet at Indiana University. I was devastated that we fell far short of expectations in the first session of competition. I tried my best Knute Rockne and Vince Lombardi impersonations to get them fired up but to no avail. After two disappointing sessions, I was at a loss as to how to respond. In an act of desperation, I promised that I would treat anyone who achieved their performance goals to a session at the pinball arcade near the hotel after the meet. I was shocked and amazed at the response to this incentive—they swam lights out. You would think that the payoff for endless hours of preparation and the blood, sweat, and tears associated with that preparation would be more than sufficient motivation to elicit personal best performances. You would think! This experience taught me not just the value of incentives but also the value of using incentives that the people you are trying to motivate can relate to. In other words, it is important to react to the reality of the situation, not necessarily to the situation as you think it should be.

For three years, our focus was exclusively on making the nationals (achieving the national championship qualifying times). After achieving that goal, we arrived at our first national championship competition with great anticipation and enthusiasm. The results were very disappointing. After many hours of soul searching to determine what had gone wrong, it occurred to me that we had already achieved our stated goal before we arrived at the competition. From that time forward, we never again talked about making the nationals. Our exclusive focus was shifted to performance at the nationals. This simple change of mindset made all the difference.

My first USA National Team coaching staff appointment was due to the performances of two of my young swimmers, Mary T. Meagher and Lisa Buese, who were selected to represent the USA on the 1979 Pan American Games team. Mary T. and Lisa were the youngest swimmers on the team, and I was the youngest, most inexperienced coach on the staff. Our training regimen was very different and more challenging than that of the other athletes on the team. When these differences became apparent, Mary T. and Lisa began to question the validity of our training plan. I attempted to convince them that we needed to trust in our plan and stay the course. Mary T. established her first of several world records in that competition (she went on to become the most accomplished female butterfly swimmer in the history of our sport), and Lisa finished a touch behind the American record holder for a silver medal in her event. Subsequent years of coaching experience taught me that even more important than the plan itself is the degree to which the team members buy in and trust the plan.

The first coaching staff meeting at that same competition taught me another valuable lesson. There was a very heated disagreement and no consensus about a certain aspect of our preparation. I was concerned that this dissension would be disruptive to our team effort. My concern was needless. After the head coach made the decision and we left the room, you would never have known that half of the coaches were adamantly opposed to that decision. All the coaches supported it without compromise or hesitation. In my opinion, this unity, loyalty, and unconditional support was the key to the success of the USA national team, and I made it a primary goal of every team that I coached throughout my career.

I continued to learn, sometimes the hard way, as I moved on to my next head coaching assignment with the Cincinnati Marlins. We had a big team at the regional championship competition with multiple swimmers in each race. I was doing my best to keep up with all of them, but invariably, one of them would slip through the cracks. One such occasion was the men's fifty-meter freestyle. The rules allow the athletes to swim any of the four strokes in the freestyle events, but they choose to swim the crawl stroke 99.9 percent of the time because it is the fastest of the four strokes. I forgot that I had given one of my swimmers the green light to swim the butterfly in this event. When he asked me to critique his race after he swam, I was too embarrassed to admit that I had missed his race while I was talking with some of his teammates about their races, so I proceeded to tell him about the technical deficiencies in his crawl stroke (which I was very familiar with from our daily practice sessions). He politely listened and then informed me that he had swum butterfly. I was too stunned and humiliated to respond. I learned that honesty truly is the best policy, and I never repeated that mistake again.

My tenure in Cincinnati also taught me about the importance of challenging perceived limitations. We were preparing to do a three-thousand-meter swim (crawl) for time in one of our Saturday morning workouts. Mary T. had moved to Cincinnati to prepare for the Olympics and was accustomed to swimming high volumes of butterfly in her workouts, but never anything close to three thousand meters straight. The butterfly is a physically demanding stroke, and conventional coaching wisdom determined that it had to be restricted to short distances in training. Mary T. was clearly a unique exception, but three thousand straight butterfly was well beyond any distance that she had ever attempted. I invited her to take on this challenge and told her that she could take the afternoon off if she achieved it. It didn't surprise me that she enthusiastically accepted, but it did surprise me that most of the other swimmers on the team complained that I was playing favorites and demanded the same opportunity. Fully expecting a disastrous result, I allowed them to step up to the challenge after informing them that, if they were unsuccessful, they would have to start over, swim three thousand crawl, and then return for the afternoon workout. Most of them, many of whom were not even butterfly specialists, successfully accepted the challenge. Few swimming coaches at the time would have believed that it could have been possible. This was a valuable lesson that taught us not to be restricted by perceived barriers.

My experiences at both Lakeside and Cincinnati also taught me the value of group synergy. There has been an age-old debate in our sport as to whether swimming is an individual sport or a team sport. My response has always been that it is whatever you choose it to be. Those who choose to make it an individual sport will focus on individual performance goals and isolated training plans specifically designed to cater to their individual needs. While the benefits of this type of training are obvious, it does not take into account the immense power that is generated by a group of people working together and challenging one another in the pursuit of a common goal. The levels of performance we can achieve in a challenging group environment will almost always far exceed those that we can achieve in an isolated environment. The daily battles that they faced in workouts enabled them to develop a mental toughness that served them well in competition.

Ironically, it is sometimes through our response to failure that we can make our greatest contribution to the success of the team. After months (and years) of intense training, the hay was in the barn, and we arrived at the 1980 national championships and Olympic trials with great anticipation. The first event of the meet featured one of our most dedicated and most popular swimmers who was considered an outside shot to make the Olympic team. Her performance fell well short of our expectations. When she touched the wall, my heart stopped partly because I felt so badly for her and partly because I knew her reaction could potentially derail our team effort before we even got started. Instead of sulking in her disappointment, she bit her lip, climbed out of the pool, and immediately began to cheer for her teammate in the next race. The impact of this unselfish reaction was powerful. When her teammates saw her put the team goals ahead of her personal disappointment, they responded with an even more determined effort. Her inspired teammates went on to establish three new world records, place six swimmers on the Olympic team (the most of any club) and win the overall national championship team title. An unselfish response to a disappointing performance was the catalyst that enabled all of this to happen.

The guiding principles discussed in this book are universal and transcend team, national, and even cultural boundaries. I arrived in

Australia at a time when the sport of swimming in that count[illegible] fallen in the world rankings. The Australian Institute of Sport (AI[illegible] was established by the federal government to boost the performances of the Australian teams in international competition. I was offered the opportunity to be the first head coach of the AIS swimming team. The young men and women in our program were being asked to entrust their hopes and dreams to this young Yankee coach who was asking them to step up to challenges that were different from and, in some ways, far greater than what had been asked of them in the past. It was a great leap of faith for them. Likewise, it was an intimidating challenge for me. Would the Aussies embrace my program, including the team-first concept that I was introducing? Would my coaching philosophy be effective in a somewhat different culture? To say that I was unsure of myself would have been an understatement, but I had learned that coaches can be successful even when they are unsure of themselves provided they don't APPEAR to be unsure. Apparently, I effectively disguised my uncertainty to the degree necessary to get the desired response from the athletes. Because they were willing to take this leap of faith, this first group of athletes at the AIS contributed substantially to Australia's resurgence in the world rankings in the following Olympics. It has been very gratifying to watch more than a few of them go on to become some of the most accomplished coaches in Australian and world swimming.

Approximately 20 years later I was in the twelfth year of my fourteen-year tenure as National Team Director for USA Swimming

Sydney, Australia for the 2000 Summer Olympics. … world rankings would support the claim that the … dominant swimming nation in the history of our … ia had closed the gap and had pulled dead even with us in the previous year. The momentum was clearly on Australia's side, and the Olympics were in their own backyard. Virtually everyone in the swimming world expected Australia to supplant the USA as the world's number one swimming power. Everyone, that is, except the 50 young men and women on the USA team. We were dealt a crushing blow in the first of eight days of competition. Our favored men's 4 x 100 freestyle relay, our "signature" relay, was beaten by the Aussies. It was the first time in the history of Olympic competition that we had failed to win that event. Our heads were spinning, and the celebration in Sydney that evening was comparable to the hometown celebration of a World Series or Super Bowl victory. This experience would have shattered the confidence and extinguished the enthusiasm of most other teams. It had the opposite effect on the 2000 USA team. It ignited a fire which enabled them to come roaring back to win the most medals ever won by a single nation in Olympic swimming history. "Sports Illustrated" magazine called it "the greatest team performance of all time". It could not have happened had it not been for the unconditional team-first attitude embraced by every member of that team and their refusal to succumb to adversity.

I always considered my swimmers to be a part of my family, but it wasn't until I became the coach of the Brophy East Swim Team in Phoenix, Arizona that I had an opportunity to coach my own kids. My two oldest were both collegiate swimmers at the time who trained with me during the summer break, and our third was a high school swimmer training with me throughout the year. Although I was very much looking forward to this opportunity, I knew there were some inherent risks. Would this have a positive or negative impact on team morale? Would it have a positive or negative impact on my relationship with them? I knew that I would have to go out of my way to ensure that it could not be perceived that my kids were given favored status or held to a lower standard, and they would have to be positive role models on the team. I had a reputation for being a task master and I put them to the test on a regular basis, pushing them in some ways well beyond what they had been challenged with in the past. Their response could not have been more gratifying. I had always been proud of my kids, but had it not been for this experience I would never have seen the strength of character that was evident under these circumstances. It is only in times of trial and challenge that strength of character is manifested. Our fourth kid was similarly challenged in his football program and responded with the same grit and determination, and I had an opportunity to coach my youngest at the University of Alabama, again, with the same result. Trial and challenge will build strength of character if we respond with the will to overcome and endure.

The final seven years of my coaching career were spent at the University of Alabama where it all started for me. At this last stop,

I distilled all the lessons that I had learned into what we called our three core values: attitude, character, and commitment. It all starts with attitude because if you don't get the attitude right, nothing else matters. Attitude is a choice. We can choose to focus on the positive or focus on the negative. It is also contagious. The choice we make will strongly influence those around us. Our mantra was to "keep it positive." Character is a broad value that encompasses many attributes that are prerequisites for success: sacrifice, discipline, perseverance, etc. We especially emphasized integrity and the importance of being reliable and trustworthy. We didn't all have to be best friends, but we all had to respect one another to become a successful team. There were two aspects of the third core value—commitment to preparation and commitment to team. Commitment to preparation was expected to be uncompromised and superior to the competition, and commitment to team was the glue that held it all together. The "team first" mentality, the willingness to sacrifice personal preferences for the good of the team, and the willingness to put a higher priority on team goals than on individual goals are the ingredients of a magical team experience that will bring the best out of each individual on the team. These three core values served us well during my tenure at my alma mater.

Fifty years of coaching for me encompassed ten different teams in four different countries. They have all been special experiences which have taught me many valuable lessons. The most rewarding aspect of my coaching career has been the relationships that are developed when a group of people make an uncompromised commitment to the pursuit of a challenging common goal. This is completely unrelated to the level of talent or even the level of performance that is achieved. It is all about striving to be the best that we can be and helping others to do the same. One of my favorite quotes is "Success in life is measured not by what you have gained for yourself but by what you have done for others."

The process of striving to be the best that we can be involves discipline, commitment, sacrifice, and perseverance through hardships, failures, and disappointments. Unfortunately, these attributes are not as mainstream in our society today as they were when I began my coaching career, but they continue to be and always will be essential to the pursuit of excellence and to personal growth and fulfillment. Our culture may change, but these prerequisites for success will never change. The greater the challenge, the greater the reward.

Not infrequently have I been asked by young coaches to share my thoughts about what they need to do to be successful. These are some of the things that I have suggested:

- Be yourself. Attempting to emulate the personality or style of a coach that is not a good fit for you will not lead to success.
- There is no coaching utopia. Do what you can to mitigate the negative aspects of your situation, but focus on the positive.
- Lead by example. Personify the attributes that you want to see in your athletes, beginning with commitment. It is

not reasonable to expect any of your athletes to be more committed than you.

- Establish challenging standards and expectations and hold your athletes accountable to those standards. Again, you must set the example.
- Be a motivator and a great salesperson. No matter how scientifically sound your program may be, it will not produce results if you are unable to get the necessary buy-in from your athletes. There are three prerequisites that are essential to becoming an effective motivator:
    1. Command respect through fairness, integrity, and transparency. Say what you mean and mean what you say.
    2. Bring passion and positive energy to the team effort (within your own style and personality).
    3. Demonstrate that you truly care about your athletes through your commitment to them. This is not related to coaching style or personality, but your athletes will be much more responsive if they believe that, beneath the surface, you truly care.

I have also endeavored to help young coaches understand that regardless of whether their athletes ever become great swimmers, in direct proportion to the extent to which they are committed to the pursuit of excellence, they are planting seeds that are essential to personal growth and success in all aspects of their lives that will help mold them into better people. That is what brings meaning and value to what they do and that is what should be given first consideration in all the decisions they make as coaches.

Coaching experience and life experience have both taught me the value of humility. The talent, opportunities and attributes that enable us to achieve success are all gifts from our Triune God who is the source of all that is good, including all our blessings. In my case, this includes a long list of mentors, colleagues, assistant coaches, and swimmers without whom I would not have achieved anything of significance. They have enriched my life immensely and I will always cherish the relationships we developed in our common pursuit of excellence. More importantly, I am forever indebted to my wife, Mary Jo, and my children, Brian, Lisa, David, Steven, and JJ, who have been the source of joy and inspiration in my life.

It has been a great privilege for me to have had the opportunity to work with so many of our sport's most accomplished athletes throughout my career. I have observed a remarkable degree of consistency and continuity in the attributes that have contributed to their success. These attributes are presented in the remainder of this book.

PART I

FOUNDATIONAL PRINCIPLES

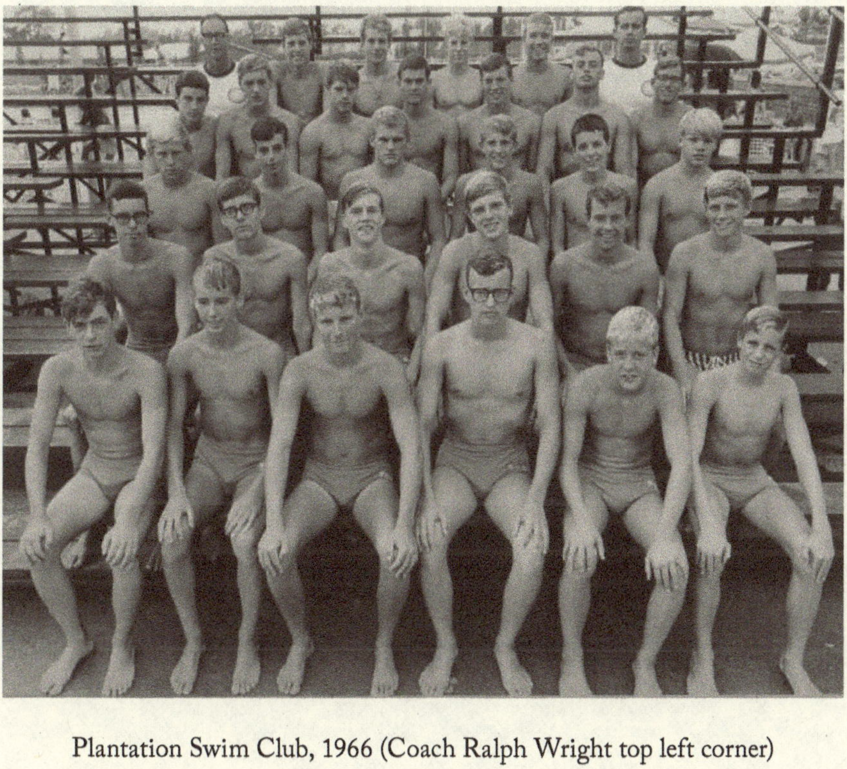

Plantation Swim Club, 1966 (Coach Ralph Wright top left corner)

Chapter 1

Priorities

Many years ago, I was watching the NFL Hall of Fame induction ceremony for one of the sport's most accomplished coaches, Tom Landry. During his acceptance speech, Coach Landry mentioned that his three priorities in life were his faith, family and football. Although I didn't think much of it at the time, after further reflection, that simple comment changed my life forever.

I was very motivated by my professional goals, but beyond that, I hadn't given much thought to my priorities in life. Coach Landry's comments prompted me to give some serious thought to this idea. Although I had to put swimming in place of football, I eventually decided that my priorities were similar to his. The life-changing part of this thought process came when I realized that these priorities were not always reflected in my daily thoughts, words, and actions. This obviously made no sense. I was then confronted with the choice of changing my lifestyle to reflect my stated priorities or changing my stated priorities to reflect my lifestyle. I chose the former.

What does this have to do with the pursuit of excellence? In my opinion, it has everything to do with it. Presumably, performance excellence is one of the top priorities of every world class athlete. We all know that performance excellence in any challenging endeavor at the world-class level requires an uncompromised commitment. It is important that we examine every aspect of our lifestyle in light of our priorities. Do you consistently apply yourself to your training sessions to the best of your ability? Do you focus on the "little things" that can make a big difference in your quest for perfection? Is your lifestyle outside of the pool compatible with performance excellence? If the answer to these questions is yes, you are on the road to success. If it is no, like I once did, you too have a big decision to make. There is no better time than now to make that decision.

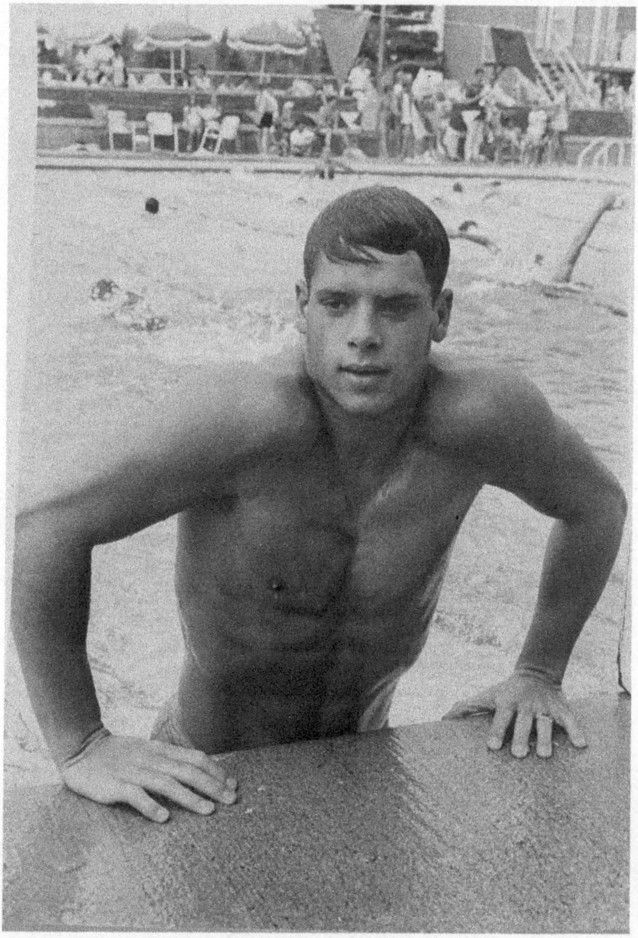

Dennis Pursley, 1967 All American

Chapter 2

Commitment

There are no shortcuts to success. Everyone wants to succeed, but not everyone is willing to make the commitment necessary to do so. When we are tempted to settle for less than our best, it might help to remind ourselves that at least some of our competitors are willing to make any sacrifice and pay any price to climb the mountain. If we are to reach the top of the mountain, we must be willing to do the same. Yes, we all have other priorities and obligations in life (faith, family, friends, and academic pursuits), but we must find ways to fulfill these obligations without compromising the pursuit of our goals.

Too often, our focus is restricted to short-term objectives. Unfortunately, the preparation strategy that is necessary to achieve the best results in the short term may not be the strategy that is required for the best results in the long run. Of course, there are always exceptions, but generally speaking, the training focus in the first half of the season should be on laying the aerobic base foundation then shifting to a greater emphasis on race-specific training in the second half. In some cases, this could involve sacrificing performance results early in the season to obtain better results when they count the most, but this is the kind of planning that is essential to long-term success.

Quite a number of years ago, I remember seeing on the pool deck at championship meets the slogan "We work harder" on the backs of T-shirts. As the years passed, hard work seemed to fall out of fashion, and those T-shirts were replaced with others that said "We work smarter, not harder." My years of experience have convinced me that we need to work smarter AND harder if we are to achieve our full potential. Although attributes such as commitment, discipline, perseverance, and sacrifice may not be as popular in our culture today as they perhaps once were, they are still every bit as essential to success. So let us acknowledge the value of these attributes, and together let us embrace them and begin the climb to the top.

Chapter 3

The Positive Choice

Every successful coach understands the importance of creating a positive training environment. Our thoughts, choices, and decisions will be influenced by the environment around us. A commitment to excellence is extremely difficult to sustain even under the best of circumstances. It becomes almost impossible to sustain if we are surrounded by negative influences or by those that promote self-indulgence or mediocrity.

As much as we are able, we should immerse ourselves in an environment that is conducive to the pursuit of excellence. This means that we should make a conscious effort to choose our friends from among those who are striving to be the best they can be and who are willing to make the necessary commitment to achieve that goal. It means that the books we read and our entertainment choices should be inspiring and challenging. Most importantly, we should challenge ourselves to keep it positive in all our thoughts, words, and actions. The closer we come to achieving this objective, the more likely we will achieve performance excellence.

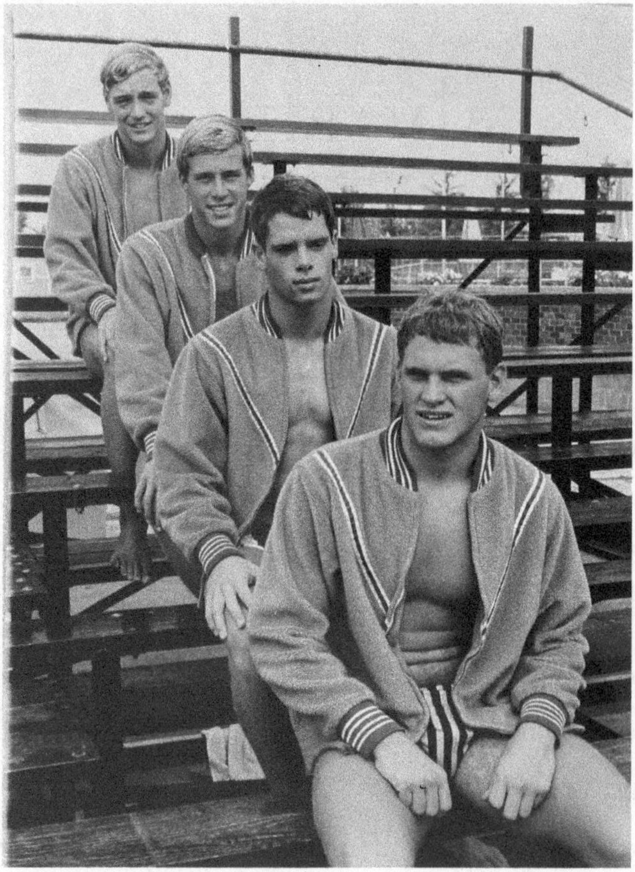

From bottom:

Bill Pocock; Dennis Pursley; Ralph (Sonny) Wright Jr; Bob Wilson;

Plantation Swim Club

national record breaking medley relay,

1968

Chapter 4

Unconditional Support

Unconditional support is one of the fundamental prerequisites of a successful team effort. This concept, however, is sometimes questioned by those who believe that authority should be challenged and that individual rights should trump team goals. While there is a time and a place for everything, the willingness to commit to a *team* effort is a foundational principle that has been the cornerstone of almost all group achievements of significance in the history of humanity. Our challenge is to determine when and how to work for change and when to fully support the team effort.

There is a time to analyze, evaluate, and constructively criticize, but if we are to become the perfect team, there also comes a time when we must set aside our personal preferences and personal agendas for the sake of the group effort. In other words, there comes a time when we must pledge our unconditional support. This principle is fundamental to the ultimate team experience in any field of endeavor.

We've all heard many times that "there is more than one way to skin a cat." Each of us would likely do things differently if our preference was always available to us. The degree of success of a group effort is determined not so much by the group approach to the task at hand as it is by the extent to which that approach is supported by each member of the group. Conditional support (i.e., "I'll support it on the condition that I agree with it") will never be as successful as unconditional support (i.e., "I'll support it and make it work for the team whether it suits me or not").

Our goal has always been to make the team experience an experience of a lifetime for each athlete who participates; an experience that provides for the achievement of individual *and* team goals. The team aspect will add a whole new dimension to this experience and will bring out the best of each individual. When a person willingly sacrifices individual privileges for the sake of the team, the experience becomes much more fulfilling and meaningful than it could have otherwise been. The team accomplishments become as gratifying and rewarding as the personal accomplishments and the benefits will more than compensate for the sacrifices that are required to achieve them.

Chapter 5

Response to Adversity

One of the few things that we can be certain of in life is that sooner or later, we will find ourselves face to face with adversity. It cannot be avoided, and it will often make or break us. Adversity is sometimes encountered in circumstances over which we have no control. When this form of adversity is presented to the entire field of competitors, we can actually make it our ally rather than our enemy. Long lines, transportation problems, uncomfortable temperatures, overcrowded conditions, etc. will often distract and discourage our competitors. If we can maintain our focus and composure in these situations, we will likely be advantaged over the competition. When circumstances beyond our control prevent us from proceeding as planned, we must be able to "roll with the punches" and modify our plans with a positive attitude and without complaint.

Adversity can also present itself in the form of failure. Here again, this is an unplanned component of the pursuit of excellence that cannot be avoided. I have heard more than a few coaches say they learn much more from failure than from success. The natural inclination for most people is to respond to failure with diminished confidence and enthusiasm. Conversely, great athletes will turn a negative into a positive by learning from the experience and responding with greater determination to succeed. We must not only be able to deliver a punch, but we must also be able to take one and bounce back strong. "Our greatest glory is not in never failing but in rising every time we fall."

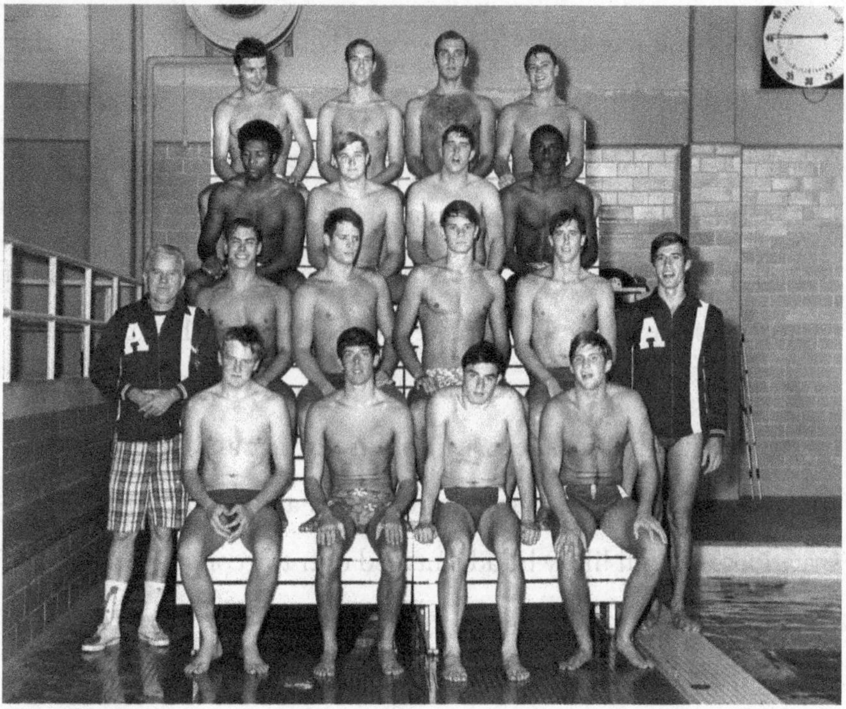

University of Alabama, 1970 (w/ Coach John Foster)

PART II

COMMITMENT TO PREPARATION

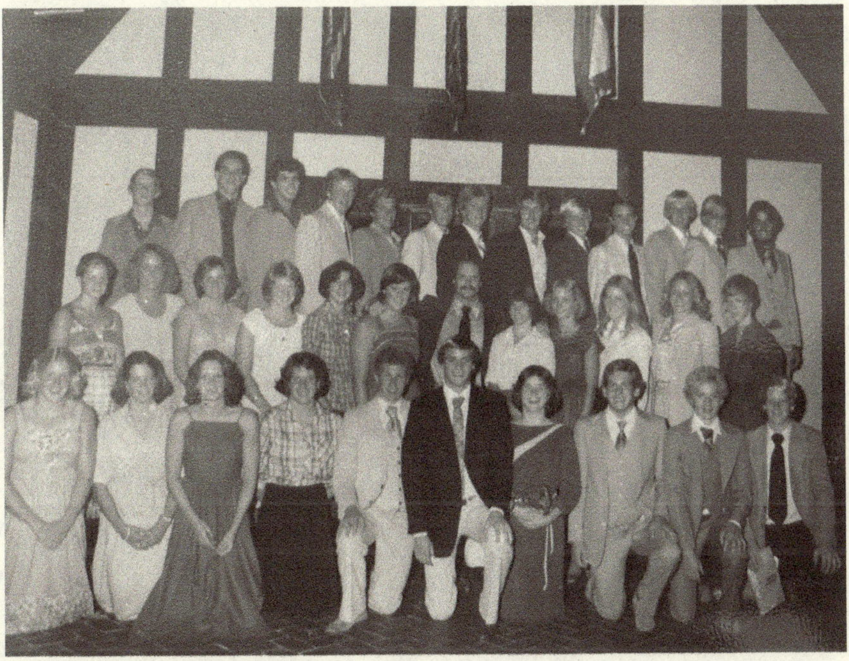

Lakeside Swim Team, 1976

Chapter 6

Expect to Be Challenged

By definition, we must be different if we want to be exceptional. This difference should manifest itself in many ways—level of commitment, attention to detail, response to adversity, willingness to sacrifice - the list goes on. One of the most important differences among those who are exceptional in any endeavor is the desire to be challenged in the pursuit of excellence. Most people avoid a challenge when possible. Instead, they prefer to live life in the comfort zone. Life in the comfort zone is a life of mediocrity. It is through responding to challenges in a positive way that we acquire the strength of character necessary to achieve excellence.

Unfortunately, it is not unusual to hear the comment, "I hope we don't have a hard workout today." An athlete who expects to be challenged or, better yet, demands to be challenged in his or her daily preparation will be advantaged over most of the competition.

When an entire team embraces challenge in this way, miracles can happen. The tedium of endless hours of practice is transformed into an invigorating, exciting, and fulfilling experience. There are few experiences more gratifying than being a part of a group effort that successfully responds to a formidable challenge.

Whether in training preparation or in major competition, it is important that we expect to be challenged, that we look forward to the challenge and that we give all that we have to give in response to that challenge. To shy away from challenge is to accept mediocrity. To be the best that we can be, we must be different.

Chapter 7

The Comfort Zone Trap

Several years ago, at a coaches' conference, one of the presenters made a statement that has stuck with me ever since. I have forgotten his name and the theme of his presentation, but I still remember this simple phrase that has had a lasting effect on my life: "The best choice is usually the most difficult choice." This little secret has been discovered by everyone who has achieved significant levels of success in any field of endeavor.

The natural inclination for most of us is to seek our comfort zone, to shy away from new and unfamiliar challenges. Personal growth, however, is attained precisely through challenging ourselves to step out of our comfort zone in pursuit of our goals. If we fail to do this, we are unlikely to experience progress, success and fulfillment. Although we all long for it, a comfortable life is rarely a productive life.

There are endless applications of this principle in the many choices and decisions we make regarding our involvement with competitive swimming—the level of commitment that we are willing to make to training preparation and a healthy lifestyle, the challenge to respond to the alarm clock on a dark and cold winter morning, our reaction to a training set that requires us to step up to a higher level of performance, the challenge to conform to team protocol when it deviates from our personal preferences to name a few.

If we are to realize our full potential as a team and as individuals, we must constantly be on guard against falling into the comfort zone trap. Are we willing to do whatever it takes (consistent with our values and moral principles) to achieve the desired result? Rather than base our choices and decisions on our personal preferences and natural inclinations, we must base them on their relationship to our goals and aspirations. More often than not, these are the most difficult choices and decisions.

Chapter 8

Just for the Heck of It!

A required set for all the swimmers in one of our national team camps was a three-thousand-meter swim for time. While this may have been a routine set for some of the distance swimmers, it was a shock to the system for the sprinters. In the age of race-specific training, many would argue that there was no purpose or benefit for the sprinters to do that kind of a set. I disagree.

While I certainly appreciate the value and necessity of race-specific training, I also believe that nonspecific training still has an important role to play in the pursuit of our goals. If our workouts consist exclusively of one type of training, no matter how significant it may be, the physiological response to that training will eventually become stale and blunted, resulting in a performance plateau. To avoid this, it is important to routinely introduce a different and fresh stimulus to the training regimen. The concept of energy system specific training (versus race specific) makes sense to me as well. The idea here is to isolate the individual energy systems involved in a given race and to design training sets that will optimally develop those systems.

What is often lost in the nonspecific versus specific debate, however, is the impact of training on confidence, psychology, and mental toughness. Many times over the years, after a breakthrough performance, I have heard one of my swimmers give credit to the "20 x 500 on 6:00" or the "10,000 for time" or the "120,000-meter peak week" for the confidence needed to prevail in the race several months later. (Just for the record, I am not recommending these sets for our sprinters.) Anytime we step out of our comfort zone to take on a challenge above and beyond the norm, we become mentally stronger, and this enhanced mental toughness will serve us well when we are confronted with the competitive challenge in our races.

I am certain that most of our sprinters would have preferred not to do the three thousand for time in the national team camp. However, to their credit, they accepted the challenge without complaint and aggressively applied themselves to the task at hand. Afterward, it was apparent that some of them surprised themselves, and they finished the session with a little extra swagger that they didn't have before. Again, I am not suggesting that these kinds of sets should be a part of the weekly training regimen, but sometimes there are significant intangible benefits to taking on a new and different challenge just for the heck of it.

CHAPTER 9

Sacrifice

In our modern, self-indulgent western culture, the title word of this chapter is sometimes regarded as an unpleasant and undesirable element of our lives. In fact, it seems that one of the goals of many people in our world today is to avoid sacrifice or minimize it as much as possible. This is unfortunate because success in school, sport, business, and in almost every other aspect of our lives is dependent upon sacrifice. Sacrifice is essential to positive and productive relationships in family life, social life, and professional life. It is largely through sacrifice that all accomplishments of significance have been achieved, both those that are recorded in the history books and the many that go unnoticed in our everyday lives. It should come as no surprise then that sacrifice is also essential to the success of a world-class athlete.

The necessity of sacrifice is readily apparent in the daily regimen of each swimmer. Generally speaking, the greater the level of sacrifice, the greater the level of success. A positive effect on performance and fulfillment can be achieved through a unified team environment. It is only through sacrifice that this environment can be established. This is often required in the form of sacrificing our personal preferences to comply with or conform to team protocol. When team protocol and policy require behavior or commitment that is not consistent with our normal routine, this can be especially difficult.

The good news is that sacrifice is not a one-way street. Whenever we sacrifice for a worthy cause or goal, the benefits almost always exceed the cost. This kind of sacrifice will enhance the performance of the team and of every individual on the team. It will also make the competitive experience significantly more rewarding and fulfilling. Even more importantly, whenever we sacrifice for a worthy cause, it serves to strengthen our character and diminish our self-centered tendencies. This in turn will enhance performance in every aspect of our lives. Once we understand and internalize this way of thinking, rather than perceive sacrifice to be an undesirable aspect of our lives, we will embrace it as an opportunity and means to achieve success and fulfillment.

Chapter 10

Perseverance

Often during my coaching career, I have been struck by the many formidable obstacles that coaches and swimmers have had to contend with: injuries, illness, disappointing performances, relationship issues, and other personal problems. At times, these obstacles can seem to be overwhelming and very discouraging, but it has been inspirational to witness the perseverance demonstrated by great athletes in responding to these challenges. As inspiring as it may be, I suppose it should not be surprising since perseverance is a key component of success.

Obstacles are inescapable in life. We can mitigate or minimize them if we live our lives with prudence and integrity, but we cannot avoid them completely. If we had a choice, I'm sure most of us would prefer not to be confronted by them. Ironically though, they are indispensable to our personal growth and to the pursuit of excellence.

It is through encountering and persevering through obstacles that we develop the strength of character necessary to achieve anything of significance. In this sense, obstacles can actually be opportunities to grow. It is also precisely because of our perseverance through these obstacles that our achievements are meaningful and rewarding. The more difficult the challenge, the more fulfilling the accomplishment. An accomplishment that is not difficult to achieve is usually not one of much value.

It may not be possible to single out one attribute that is the single most important in achieving success in any endeavor, but perseverance is certainly as important as any other. It is one of the fundamental prerequisites in the successful pursuit of our goals.

The following words of wisdom more effectively reflect these thoughts:

- To endure is greater than to dare; to tire out hostile fortune; to be daunted by no difficulty; to keep heart when all have lost it—who can say this is not greatness? —William Thackeray
- Our greatest glory is not in never falling, but in rising every time we fall. —Confucius
- Ask not for victory, ask for courage. For if you can endure, you bring honor to us all; even more, you bring honor to yourself. —from the Decathlon
- He conquers who endures. —Persius

- The ultimate measure of a man (athlete) is not where he stands in times of comfort and convenience, but where he stands at times of challenge.
- No man is a failure until he gives up.
- The highest reward for a person's toil is not what they get for it, but what they become by it. —John Ruskin
- So stick to the fight when you're hardest hit; it's when things seem worse that you must not quit.

Chapter 11

Mental Toughness Is a Habit

There is little dispute that mental toughness is a key component of competitive success. Sometimes, however, we make the mistake of believing that we will respond to a challenge with mental toughness when really needed, but we need not be concerned about it in all other situations. We plan to rise to the occasion on the main set each day but are content to train in our comfort zone on the other sets. Or we may expect to successfully respond to the challenge in major competition, but we are content to settle for less than our best in less significant competitions. If we take this approach to preparation, we will likely be disappointed with the end result.

Aerobic fitness, anaerobic fitness, stroke efficiency, strength and power, and every other component of race preparation must be gradually developed through countless repetitions in training. Mental toughness is no different. It will likely fail us when it really counts if it has not become a habit. When faced with a major challenge, we will most often revert back to our habitual tendencies.

We all know of athletes who personify this attribute. They seem to give 110 percent to everything they do in training and competition. They make no distinction between the main sets and the other sets, the major competition and the other competitions, their best events or their other events, their good days or their bad days. Regardless of the circumstances, they always race tough. Through habitual reinforcement, mental toughness becomes an ingrained part of who they are. These are the athletes who will almost always win the close races. These are the athletes who will almost always perform well under pressure. These are the athletes whom we should all strive to emulate.

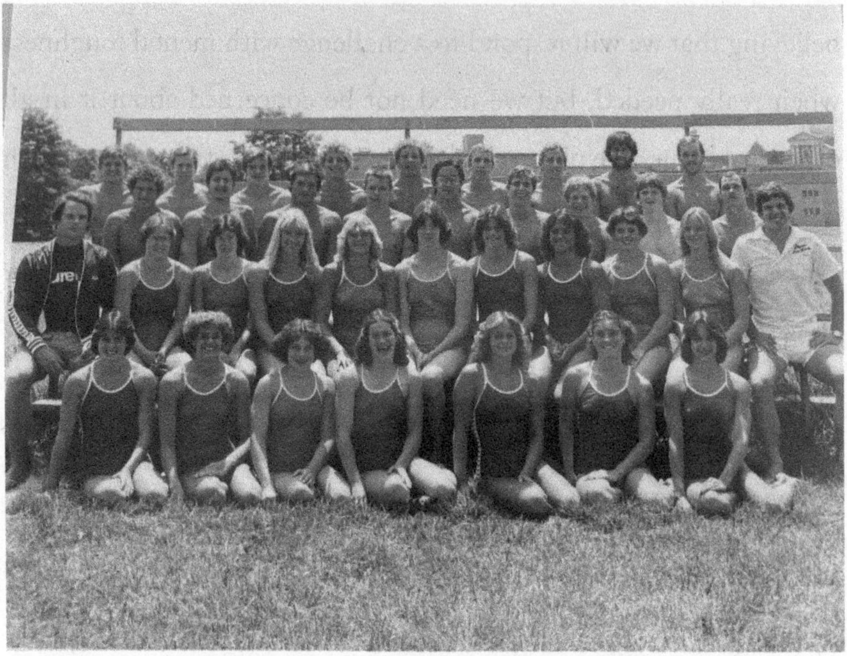

Cincinnati Marlins 1980 National Champions

Chapter 12

The Pack Mentality

The sport of swimming has evolved in many different ways over the decades. One of the most noticeable changes in the daily training environment has been a gradual shift from a group approach to training to more of an individual approach. In many cases, the pendulum has swung from one extreme to the other. Since both approaches offer obvious benefits, it seems to me that a combination of both would produce the best results.

The benefits of an individual approach to training are obvious. A program designed to address the individual needs and unique physiology of each swimmer certainly makes sense. However, mental toughness and competitive instincts are also important to success in any sport. Just as technical race skills are developed through constant repetition in training, so too are competitive instincts. The group approach to training can more effectively facilitate the development of these attributes.

I have been fortunate more than once in my career to have had the opportunity to coach a large group of highly competitive swimmers, both at the developmental and world-class levels of our sport. On these occasions, the aggressive pack mentality that evolved in these groups served to enhance race toughness and to push each individual in the group to levels of performance beyond what they would have achieved on their own. It should be no surprise that a competitive environment will bring the best out of a competitive athlete.

This same pack mentality can enhance the performance of each individual on the team in major competition. Athletes will be motivated by, and feed off of, the successes of one another. The desire to compete and to respond aggressively to the challenge becomes contagious. It is this group dynamic that produces the greatest team performances in any sport.

Although the individual approach to training has much to offer and is here to stay, it does not have to be used exclusively. There is a time and a place for everything. The individual approach integrated with the group approach will give us the best of both worlds—physiologically enhanced preparation combined with stronger competitive instincts and mental toughness. An emphasis on both will better ensure that an athlete will step up rather than give up when confronted with a competitive challenge.

Chapter 13

Little Things Make a Big Difference

We have often heard the saying "little things make a big difference," and there is much truth to this statement in sport. Technical efficiency in starts, turns, and finishes often determines who wins the race. Minor adjustments in stroke technique will sometimes have a major impact on performance results. Especially at the elite level of performance, the "little things" will frequently make the difference between success and failure. Too often, it is these important "little things" that are neglected or overlooked altogether.

Many of us are inclined to focus all our attention on the major events, opportunities, and challenges in our lives. We tell ourselves that what really matters is to rise to the occasion when it really counts, and that the little things are insignificant and unimportant. There are two major flaws in this line of thinking. Firstly, for most of us, the major events and opportunities are few and far between. The mundane daily routine (i.e., the little things) comprises 99 percent of our lives. In this respect, it is the little things that determine who we are as athletes and as people. If we restrict our best efforts to the major events, we will fall well short of our potential.

Secondly, it is precisely through committing our best efforts to the little things that we better prepare ourselves for success when confronted with the major challenges in life, both because these little things do in fact make a big difference and because our best effort becomes a part of who we are if we apply it on a daily basis. To be the best that we can be in everything that we do is to live life to the fullest extent. Why settle for anything less?

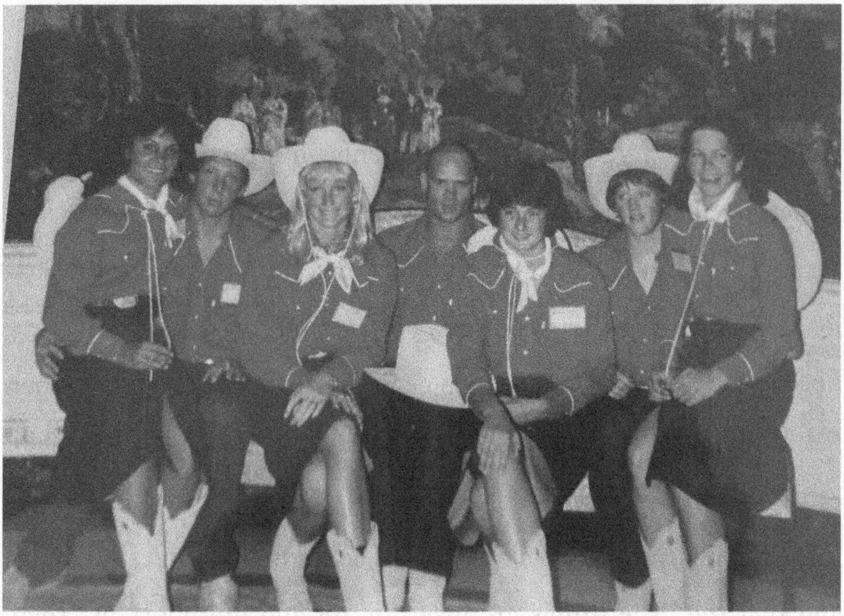

Stephanie Elkins; Bill Barret; Kim Carlisle; Dennis Pursley;
Mary T Meagher; Glenn Mills; Lisa Buese
1980, Cincinnati Marlins Olympians

PART III

PERFORMANCE EXCELLENCE

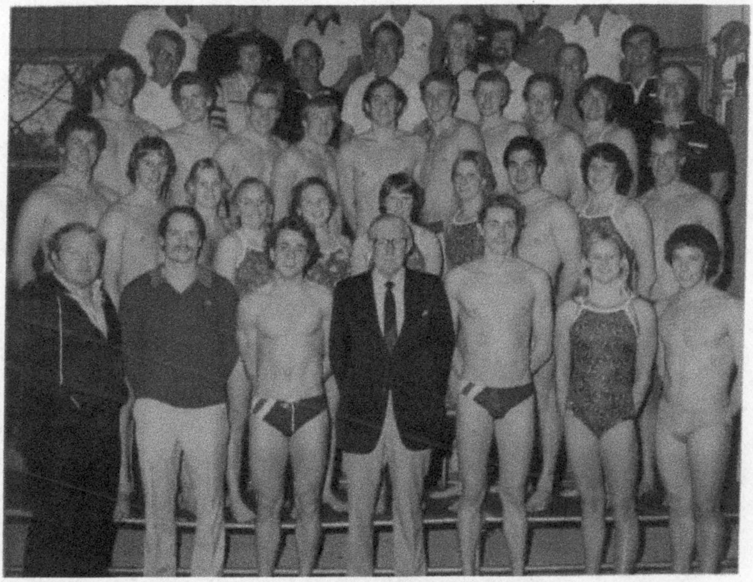

Australian Institute of Sport, 1982

Chapter 14

When Opportunity Knocks

Our biggest regrets in life are often related to the failure to recognize and take advantage of the opportunities that come our way. When opportunity presents itself, will we be prepared to take full advantage of it? In my opinion, the answer to this question will be determined by the degree to which we accomplish the following objectives:

1. Superior Preparation

Everyone will bring talent to the blocks in championship competition. Talent alone will not win medals or even enable us to swim personal best times. In most cases, to swim faster than our competition, we will have to be better prepared. We need to remind ourselves of this simple fact when we are tempted to take shortcuts or to settle for less than our best. We must adopt a whatever-it-takes attitude and be willing to go above and beyond the commitment that our competitors are making in our preparation for success.

2. Healthy Lifestyle

Although training for peak performance in championship competition is far more challenging, maintaining a healthy lifestyle can be equally important to success. Illness and injury will not necessarily prevent us from achieving our goals (we all know of athletes who have successfully rebounded from serious injury or illness), but they can diminish the probability of success. Extra attention to healthy lifestyle choices, such as dressing appropriately in the winter, healthy diets, getting plenty of rest, and developing healthy personal hygiene habits could very possibly determine whether or not you achieve your championship goals.

3. Building Confidence

As Henry Ford once said, "Whether you think you can or think you can't, you are probably right." Doubts and negative thoughts will creep into our conscious mind from time to time, but it is important that we recognize them for what they are—thoughts, not reality. Beneath these negative thoughts, we must believe that we are capable of accomplishing our goals. Most importantly, we must believe that we belong on the big stage and that we are ready to successfully compete with anyone.

4. Handling Pressure

We can expect the public and media attention to be turned up to a fever pitch in the weeks and even months preceding the championship competition. Will we be distracted and become unglued by all this pressure, or will we be prepared to handle it effectively or, better yet, be prepared to use it to our advantage? We will need to tap into this positive energy and enjoy the experience. The ability to "go with the flow" and "roll with the punches" will also serve us well in pressure situations.

5. Team-First Culture

A strong team culture cannot be attained without the willingness to sacrifice personal preferences for the sake of the team. The team is important to all of us, but not everyone is willing to make it the highest priority when it conflicts with individual preferences. This sometimes requires a leap of faith, but the performance enhancing and overall experience enhancing benefits can be immense if we are willing to take it.

All of the above are basic prerequisites for success. Although plain and simple, these objectives can only be accomplished with a strong will, discipline, perseverance, and willingness to sacrifice.

Chapter 15

Self-Reliance and Adaptability

Most national federations and elite programs endeavor to provide their swimmers with sophisticated support, services, and resources which are designed to optimize and enhance performance at the highest levels. Our sport has progressed dramatically in this area in recent years. Sport science support includes soft tissue massage, race analysis information, biomechanical filming and analysis, tracking of physiological data, specialized strength and conditioning coaching, nutritional guidance, sport psychology support, and lifestyle counseling. Support staff commit countless hours of service and large sums of money to provide the ideal environment in which to train and compete. Nothing is left to chance.

Only a few short years ago, this level of support was nonexistent in our sport. Support for swimmers consisted exclusively of a coach and an overcrowded pool, often available only at inconvenient hours.

While the commitment required of today's world-class competitor certainly deserves all the support that is currently provided, there is a potential downside to all these benefits. We must guard against the inclination to become overly dependent upon this support for performance results. Regardless of the extremes that we may go to in an effort to control the environment, there will inevitably come a time when we will be confronted with obstacles that we cannot control even with our best efforts. The self-reliant and adaptable athlete will be advantaged in these situations.

We can all think of inspiring examples of great accomplishments that were achieved under the worst of circumstances. A self-reliant athlete will rise to the occasion when faced with obstacles while others may tend to succumb to them and use them as excuses for subpar performances. It is important that we accept full responsibility for our performances, both successful and unsuccessful. By doing so, we will retain control of those performances rather than putting ourselves at the mercy of the circumstances.

If we simultaneously pursue both objectives of exploiting the benefits of advanced technology but not becoming dependent upon this technology, we will be advantaged in the face of adversity. Success will be assured whether because of or in spite of the circumstances.

Chapter 16

Stepping Down to the Big Meet

We all know that unfamiliarity can sometimes result in intimidation, which in turn can adversely affect performances. Carefully planned physical and mental preparation can minimize intimidation and enable us to make the most of the opportunities that come our way.

It is important to anticipate well in advance the physiological stresses that will likely be encountered in peak performance competition. How many events will you likely swim (including relays)? How much recovery time will you likely have between events and sessions? These scenarios should be replicated in the training program and in the prep meets so they won't be unfamiliar in the championship meet. It can also be helpful to take it one step further by subjecting yourself to greater challenges in preparation than you expect to face in the championship meet so that you will not only be familiar with the championship meet scenario, but it will actually be a step down from what you have experienced in preparation.

It is also important to anticipate the logistical challenges that may be encountered. How long will it take to get to the pool from the hotel, how much walking will be involved, how much rest will you have between heats and finals, and what meal options will be available to you? (In some cases, it may be necessary to stock your hotel room with nutritional food and drink.) Here again, it is better to anticipate the worst-case scenarios and rehearse your plans to successfully respond to them.

Effective mental preparation is perhaps the best strategy that we can use to eliminate the fear factor caused by intimidation. It is difficult, if not impossible to replicate the energy and excitement of some championship meets, but effective mental preparation can enable us to respond in a positive way to this environment so that it can be utilized to enhance our performances rather than to suppress them. Confidence and enthusiasm results from knowing that we are well prepared to make adversity our ally and to respond in a positive way to all challenges, both foreseen and unforeseen.

It is also helpful to keep things in perspective and to remember that with every opportunity, we have everything to gain and nothing to lose. Your personal best time can never get any slower, it can only stay the same or get faster. Well-prepared, confident, and optimistic athletes will look forward to the championship opportunity and will tap into the positive energy of a big meet to lift their performances. This kind of preparation will enable us make the most of the unique and exciting opportunities that come our way.

Chapter 17

A Balanced Perspective

Most people would probably agree that it's not a good thing to underestimate the strength of the competition and that we can sometimes set ourselves up for failure with overconfidence or an overly inflated ego. Performance can also be negatively impacted by underestimating your own accomplishments and abilities. Successful swimmers will recognize both their strengths and weaknesses (we all have them) and will develop strategies to capitalize on the former and minimize the latter. They draw confidence from their accomplishments and are motivated to eliminate their shortcomings. A balanced perspective is important to the process of becoming the best that you can be.

It can be beneficial to look to those who are ahead of us. The desire to emulate them (and chase them) can help bring the best out of us. It is also important to occasionally look back and see how far we have come. Rookies and lower-seeded swimmers in major competitions can sometimes feel overwhelmed and out of place, but nothing could be further from the truth. The pecking order myth is one that is shattered in every major competition by rookies, and other swimmers in early heats who refuse to concede that the results are predetermined by the pre-race rankings.

Whether we're talking about the sectional championships or Olympic games, it is important to feel like you belong, to look forward to the challenge, and to enjoy the experience. It is equally important to avoid the temptation to be satisfied with participation without regard to performance. This is not likely to happen in a trials competition, but I have often seen it happen in major international competitions. Successful *performance* is the goal, not participation. What is successful performance? It has nothing to do with the place you finished or even how fast you swam. It has everything to do with how close you came to swimming up to the best of your ability on that day. Circumstances beyond your control may not allow you to swim as fast as you would like to swim, but *no* circumstances can prevent you from being focused, determined, and aggressive in your racing. If your *effort* has left nothing to be desired, you can be proud of your performance.

The great athletes are rewarded by success and motivated, rather than discouraged, by failure. They learn from their mistakes and turn bad into good whether in the next race, the next meet, or the next season. Whether you are a rookie or a veteran, the ingredients for success are the same:

- Appreciate the opportunity
- Enjoy the experience
- Expect the best (give yourself a chance)
- Accept the responsibility to perform (regardless of the circumstances)
- Confront adversity with confidence and determination
- Give it your best shot
- Contribute in every way that you can to the success of the team

Chapter 18

Performing Under Pressure

We have all experienced pressure. Do we welcome it, or do we dread it? The answer to that question will likely have much to do with our performance results. Pressure will almost always impact performance. The way in which we respond to it will determine whether it is a positive or a negative impact.

Pressure can come from outside sources or from within ourselves. We must learn to control it, or it will control us. If we manage it properly, pressure can be used to stimulate our adrenalin and lift our performances to a higher level. It can enhance our incentive, motivation, and determination. If we allow pressure to control us, however, it will deplete our energy and destroy our confidence.

The difference between athletes who respond well to pressure and those who don't is often a matter of perspective. Those who thrive on pressure will look at every challenge as an opportunity and will tap into the energy that is prevalent in a high-pressure environment. They will relish the spotlight and embrace the moment.

Those who are unable to handle the pressure will often associate their performance with their self-worth. They believe that their quality of life may be diminished or that they are somehow less significant or of less value as a person if they fail to achieve their performance goals. Although this mindset has no basis in reality, it can create an intimidating level of pressure that is likely to crush rather than enhance performance.

A balanced perspective that recognizes the significance of the opportunity combined with an "everything to gain and nothing to lose" attitude is the perspective that will enable an athlete to use the pressure to his or her advantage. Learning to effectively handle pressure will be as important as any other aspect of our preparation in our quest for success.

Chapter 19

Finishing Strong

It has been well-established in championship competition that the swimmers who are able to finish strong are more likely to make it to the podium than those who focus on the front end of the race, especially in the longer events. The following components of training and racing are all essential to strong finishes:

1. Aerobic Foundation

While race-specific training is of obvious importance to preparation for peak performance, a strong finish is dependent upon a good aerobic base. Threshold training should be strongly emphasized in early season training to build the base and then continued throughout the season to the extent necessary to maintain the optimum level of aerobic fitness.

2. Effective Tapering

If a solid aerobic foundation has been established, effortless race pace is achieved in the warm-up, and the race has been swum efficiently, over tapering could be the cause of failing to finish strong. In some cases, a drop taper is more effective and in others a more gradual taper will work better, but in all cases the taper must be designed to maintain peak aerobic fitness levels throughout the competition.

3. Race Strategy

From a physiological perspective, an evenly paced swim is the most energy efficient swim. The get-out-fast strategy will more often than not end up being a crash-and-burn strategy. Swimmers who are patient on the front end will have more gas in the tank at the back end.

4. Race Efficiency

On the front end of the race, more important than how fast you go is *how* you go fast. In other words, hitting your target splits is not enough. You have to hit them with maximal efficiency and minimal expenditure of effort. I often hear the comment that "it felt so easy going out." It *always* feels easy going out, but it will deteriorate on the back half if the front end of the race was inefficient (poor stroke technique, too tight, wrong tempo, too short, etc).

5. Mental Toughness

This is what racing is all about. If it comes down to the last few strokes, the swimmer who is the most determined will generally win.

It is important that all these possibilities are considered when analyzing race performances and planning for future success. There is no doubt that the swimmers who are able to finish strong will be advantaged over their competitors.

Chapter 20

No Excuses

Why is it that most champions will usually accept full responsibility for their unsuccessful performances, while many of us typically play the blame game when we don't succeed? To some extent, I believe that this is related to our natural inclinations and to who we are as athletes and as people. The willingness to accept accountability is not an insignificant attribute of a champion. Instead, it is an attribute that contributes to successful performances.

If we are inclined to make excuses for unsuccessful performances, we are in effect relinquishing control of those performances. The underlying message is that the obstacles to success cannot be overcome, and that we are unable to perform successfully in less-than-ideal circumstances.

Conversely, those who accept responsibility and accountability for their own performances are in control or their own destiny. They are confident that they will succeed whether because of or in spite of the circumstances. Circumstances that they cannot control will not diminish their confidence or distract their focus. They believe that it is within their capabilities to overcome the barriers that stand in the way of success.

Many of the most impressive and inspirational performances in the history of sport have been achieved under the worst of circumstances. Champions will respond to a greater challenge with greater determination. Adversity will bring the best out of them. Rarely will they fall short of expectations, but when they do, they will offer "no excuses."

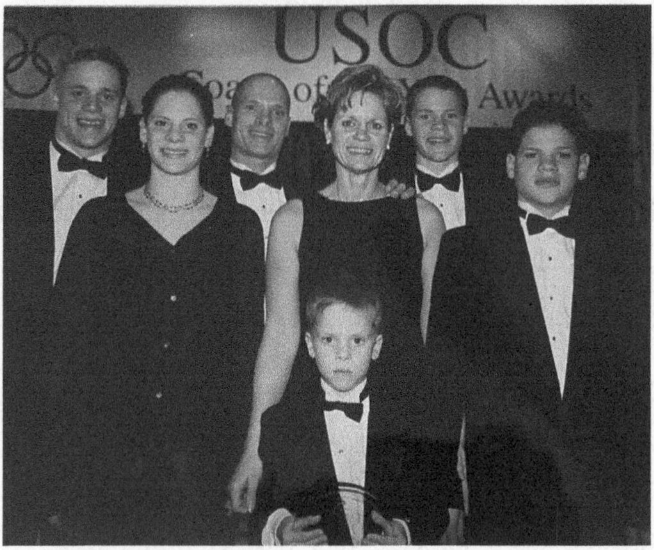

Pursley family – top row:

Brian; Lisa; Dennis; Mary Jo; David; Steven

– bottom row:

Joseph (JJ)

U.S. Olympic Committee 2000

Coach of the Year Awards

Chapter 21

Unity and Focus

Times have changed in competitive swimming. Gone forever are the days when we could wait until a few weeks before the championship competition to focus on preparation for success. It is now necessary to unite behind a strategy focused on success much further in advance and to evaluate everything we do in and out of the pool in light of its impact on performance. It is important to remind ourselves that our toughest opponents are doing the same. Their planning, training, and even their personal lives are all focused on achieving the desired results in championship competition.

Even more important than the approach we take to preparation is the extent to which we unite behind and support that approach. No program will succeed at the championship level unless it is fully supported. This applies to support for aspects of the program that don't suit our personal preferences as well as for those that do. It is this unity and unconditional support that often distinguishes the successful teams from those that fail.

Those who believe that swimming is not a team sport and that the team concept is not appropriate are missing out on one of the most powerful and rewarding aspects of participation. With strong team support, most of us can more effectively overcome the many obstacles, challenges, and frustrations that stand between us and success. Team goals, combined with individual goals, will provide twice the incentive and rewards of individual goals alone. Most of us can more easily perform up to the best of our ability in a positive and spirited team atmosphere. This is what can set us apart from our competitors.

In the competitive world of swimming today, we are faced with the challenge to respond with a higher level of unity, support, and spirit than ever before. If we meet this challenge, we will be rewarded with championship success.

CHAPTER 22

The "Team First" Mindset

The question of whether swimming is an individual sport or a team sport has been debated for decades. The answer is that it will be whatever we choose it to be. My experience has thoroughly convinced me that the team approach has the potential to be more rewarding, more fulfilling, and more successful than the individual approach. The willingness to sacrifice personal preferences for the sake of the team is an essential and fundamental prerequisite to the creation of a strong team environment. Herein lies the catch. The team is important to all of us, but not everyone is willing to make it the highest priority when it conflicts with individual preferences. Ironically, individual performances are invariably enhanced in a strong team environment. Although it sometimes requires a leap of faith that some are reluctant to make, the "team first" choice is a win-win choice. Unfortunately, we often want to have our cake and eat it too by paying lip service to the team concept but stopping short of the commitment required to make it happen.

So what are the benefits of a "team first" mindset? It will facilitate the development of a positive environment, which in turn will enhance the probability of team *and* individual success. By taking some of the focus and pressure off ourselves, it will help us to establish a balanced perspective. It provides strength to overcome. It will provide additional incentive to perform well and will make the competitive experience more rewarding and fulfilling. There are few experiences more rewarding than to be a contributing member of a successful group effort of significance.

There is a direct correlation between the degree to which we are willing to sacrifice for the team and the degree to which we receive these benefits. Sometimes, it does not occur until long after our athletic careers are finished, but at some point, most of us eventually come to the realization that the most fulfilling aspect of our athletic experience was not the achievement of our goals but the personal bonds and relationships that resulted from the sacrifices we made on behalf of our teammates and our commitment to our common mission.

PART IV

SUCCESS AND FULFILLMENT

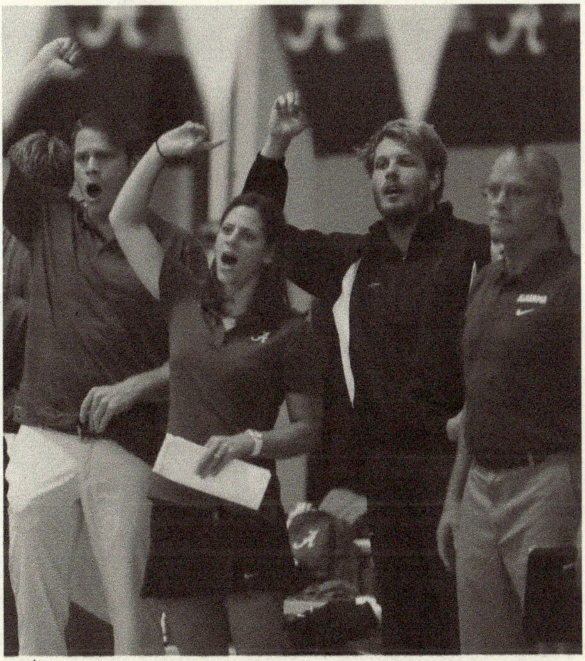

Coach David Pursley, Coach Lisa (Pursley) Ebling, Bjoern Hornikel (All American), Coach Dennis Pursley

Chapter 23

Honest Analysis

Honest analysis is a critical component of progress and success. If we are to fully develop our potential, we must be able to objectively and accurately evaluate our strengths, weaknesses, opportunities, and challenges. This requires a balanced approach to the process of evaluation, but some people tend to focus exclusively on their strengths and opportunities, while others tend to dwell on their weaknesses and challenges.

This latter approach to analysis is clearly undesirable. An inordinate preoccupation with our weaknesses and challenges can result in a lack of confidence and enthusiasm. Athletes who fall into this category will rarely, if ever, experience any gratification or fulfillment in their performances. They will struggle to find the motivation to make the daily commitment to training and will usually expect the worst in competition. This is obviously not a recipe for success.

Less obvious is the negative impact on progress that can be caused by the opposite extreme. Athletes who put their heads in the sand and fail to identify their weaknesses, or underestimate the magnitude of the challenges they face, will not likely strengthen their weaknesses or be adequately prepared for a formidable challenge. Because they see only the bright side, they will usually tend to be complacent with their performances even when they fall short of their potential. While the positive disposition of these athletes is certainly preferable to the negative perspective of the others, neither of these approaches to analysis will lead to progress or excellence.

A more balanced approach will lead to a more successful outcome. It is important to objectively identify our weakness and shortcomings and to develop a strategy to eliminate or mitigate them. Likewise, we must be willing to acknowledge when we could have done better and accept responsibility for our unsuccessful performances. At the same time, we must draw confidence from our strengths and give ourselves credit when credit is due. Most importantly, we must believe that hard work and superior preparation will enable us to achieve our goals.

This balanced approach to analysis and preparation will better ensure that we achieve our full potential.

Chapter 24

The Issue of Winning

During a half-century of involvement with competitive swimming, I have observed an interesting array of attitudes and perspectives toward the concept of winning. At one extreme, there are those who believe that a focus on winning is misdirected, unhealthy, and puts undue pressure on the competitors. These people tend to downplay the importance of performance and focus instead on the value of participation in a broad sense. They are usually intimidated by talk of medal counts and team scores. At the other extreme are those who believe that winning is everything and the only thing. They adopt a win-at-all-costs attitude and believe that "first is first, and second is last." To them, we have failed if we have achieved anything less than a gold medal or a first-place finish in the team standings regardless of the circumstances. I really don't share either of these perspectives.

It has always been my opinion that winning, in the spirit of good sportsmanship and fair play, is a worthy, noble, and honorable goal to strive for. I believe that we lose the spark that helps us to become the best that we can be when we stop trying to win, or neglect to include winning as one of our objectives. The greatest competitors and most dominant teams typically respond positively to the challenge of winning. They will enthusiastically embrace it and relish the opportunity rather than shy away from it. This challenge brings the best out of them.

My view departs from the "winning is everything" perspective, however, in the sense that I do not believe that success or failure is contingent upon achieving this goal. Heart, passion, and competitive determination are the measures of success. The key question is not whether we have won, but whether we have left no stone unturned in preparing to win and have completely spent ourselves in the *effort* to win. Theodore Roosevelt may have said it best when he said,

> "The credit belongs to the man who is actually in the arena; whose face is marred by dust and sweat and blood; who strives valiantly; who errs and comes short again and again; who knows the great enthusiasms, the great devotions, and spends himself in a worthy cause; who at the best knows in the end the triumph of high achievement; and who at the worst, if he fails, at least fails while daring greatly."

Vince Lombardi put it more succinctly when he said,

"Winning is not everything, but making the effort to win is."

How much more exciting would competition be if every competitor would step up to the blocks in every race with the intention of winning, and every team would expect to be challenged to win medals and would respond positively to that challenge, and every swimmer would want to be aware of and motivated by the team scores and medal counts, and regardless of the outcome, all our athletes could hold their heads high and experience the great intrinsic rewards that result from knowing they have given all that they have to give?

Chapter 25

We Can All Contribute

Not all of us have the talent to win medals at the highest levels of competition, but we can all contribute to the success of the team. The age group coach who is finding the time and patience to teach our future Olympians to swim, the parents who are driving them to morning workouts, the teammates who are challenging them in training, the officials who are spending their weekends running swimming meets, the admin staff who are handling all the logistics, the sport science staff who are supporting the national team, and the coaches who sacrifice weekends, holidays and any semblance of a "normal" life are all making invaluable contributions to the success of the national team. Without the top to bottom team effort, there would be no national team program and no medals for the USA swimming team.

As important as they are, however, isolated individual efforts in and of themselves will not result in the level of success that we aspire to achieve. It is equally important that we work together in a unified team effort. We will all have different opinions as to how to go about achieving any given objective, and we will all be presented with countless opportunities to support or resist the team approach. When we are willing to make personal sacrifices for the sake of the team effort, we become a formidable team. It is this kind of environment that produces gold medals and personal best performances. Each time we make the positive choice to support the team effort, we are contributing to the success of the program and everyone in it. When this happens and our objectives are accomplished, everyone involved can take special pride in their personal contributions to a job well done.

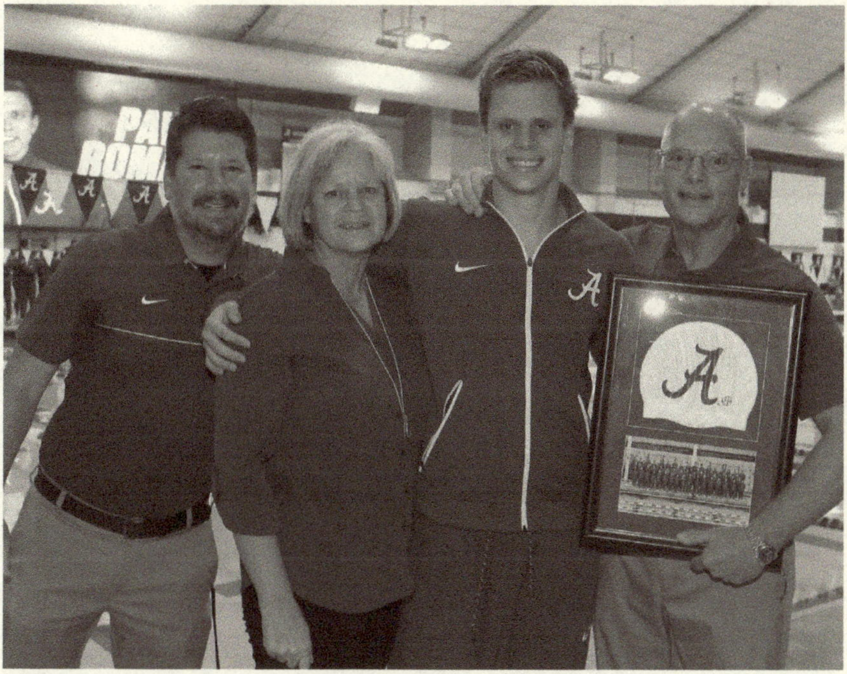

Coach James Barber, Mary Jo Pursley, Joseph (JJ) Pursley, Coach Dennis Pursley

Chapter 26

Appreciation

It is important that we occasionally remind ourselves of how privileged we are to have the opportunities that are available to us in our athletic careers. The tendency is to take them for granted, especially for the veterans who have been there and done that. If we don't appreciate an opportunity, we won't value it; if we don't value it, we won't put our heart and soul into it; if we don't put our heart and soul into it, we won't achieve the results or experience the potential rewards and benefits to the fullest degree. In other words, we will fail to take full advantage of the opportunity.

Appreciation can also help us put things in their proper perspective. In enables us to recognize the fact that much of the credit for our accomplishments and opportunities is due to those around us. Our family, friends, coaches, teachers, and teammates have all helped us become who we are, and many behind-the-scenes people we don't even know have worked hard to provide the opportunities that have been presented to us. Through appreciation, we are more grateful for what we have (which is more than most) and more inclined to make the most of it, rather than to be dissatisfied because of what we don't have. All this can help us achieve our full potential.

We all have a responsibility and an obligation to do everything we can to take full advantage of the opportunities that are presented to us. The formula for success is not complicated:

Commitment + Teamwork = Success

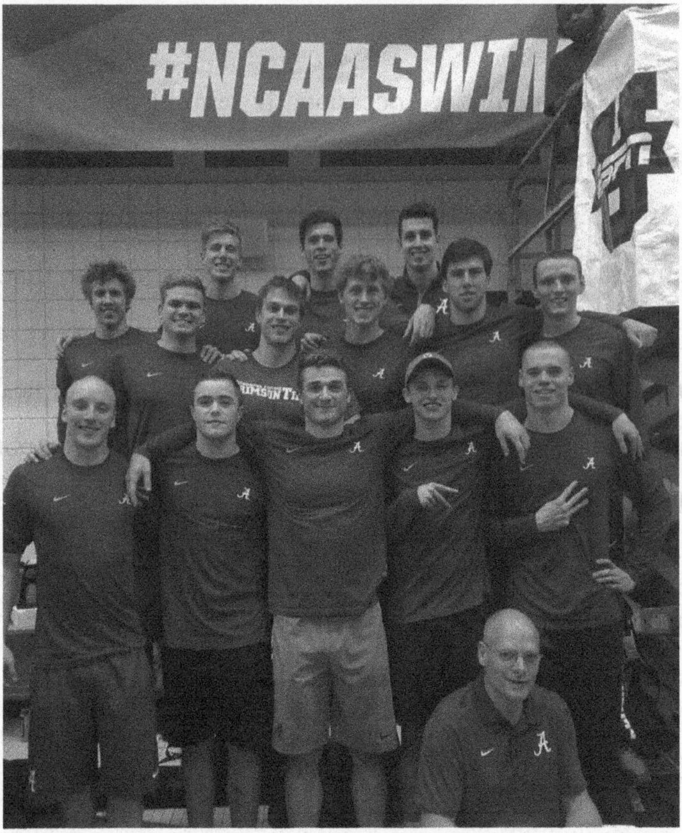

University of Alabama NCAA Championship Team, 2016

Chapter 27

The Real Value in What We Do

The fortune and fame that sometimes results from performance excellence provides those who achieve it with a platform to profoundly impact the lives of others, whether they wish this to be so or not. Their words, actions, and lifestyle will be emulated by many of their admiring fans. This is an enormous responsibility, but it is also an enormous opportunity.

By competing with good sportsmanship and respect for coaches, administrators, teammates, and fellow competitors; by personifying the values and attributes that are inherent to personal growth and achievement (appreciation, gratitude, loyalty, integrity, etc.); and by giving back and helping others to achieve success, performance excellence can be parlayed into an achievement of far greater significance than any gold medal or world record.

The most fundamental and most important responsibility of a leader is to be a good role model.

"Success in life is measured not by what we have gained for ourselves, but by what we have done for others."

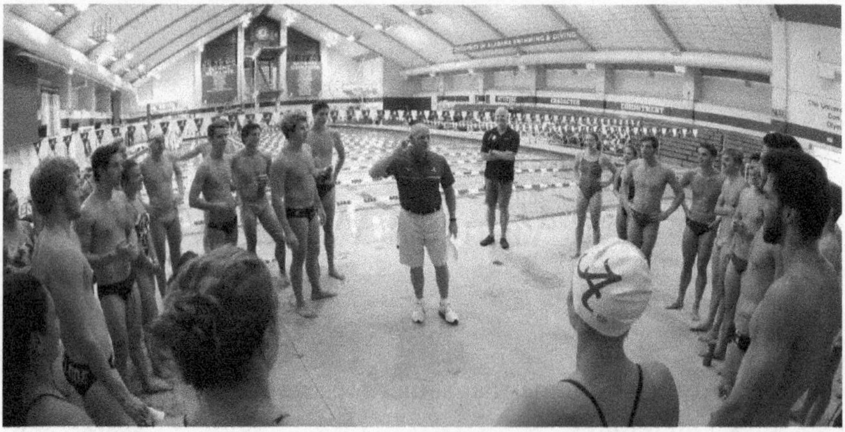

Coach Dennis Pursley with the University of Alabama Swim Team

CHAPTER 28

Attributes of a Champion

1. Recognizing Opportunity

Life is full of opportunities. Many of them come and go because we fail to recognize them. Champions will recognize the opportunities that are presented to them and will take full advantage of them.

2. Positive Attitude

- Attitude is contagious and affects the people around us.
- A positive attitude increases the probability of success; a negative attitude decreases the probability of success.

3. Attention to Detail

Detail can be mundane and tedious. A champion knows that the "little things" can make a big difference in the final result.

4. Willingness to Strengthen Our Weaknesses

Most of us are inclined to focus on our strengths and ignore our weaknesses. Champions capitalize on their strengths and focus strongly on eliminating their weaknesses.

5. Willingness to "Take It to the Limit"

Champions will test the boundaries in the pursuit of excellence.

6. Embracing a Challenge

Many people shy away from challenge. A champion will embrace it.

7. Confidence and Focus

A champion will compete with confidence and focus when others succumb to doubts and distractions.

8. Performing under Pressure

A champion will utilize pressure to enhance rather than suppress performance.

9. Positive Response to Failure and Disappointment

A champion will respond to failure and disappointment with a fighting spirit and increased determination, while others respond with shattered confidence and despondency.

10. Superior Preparation

This begins with a strong work ethic and self-discipline.

11. Uncompromised Commitment

A champion will find a way to do whatever it takes to be the best that he/she can be and avoid the things that will detract from this goal. All choices and decisions will be based on whether they will enhance or inhibit the probability of success.

12. Strength of Will

Mental toughness and competitive tenacity.

13. Staying Positive over the Long Haul

Realizing that every comment can make a difference.

14. Perseverance

In good times and in bad.

15. Handling Adversity and Overcoming Obstacles

- Resiliency, flexibility, adaptability

- "Our greatest glory is not in never failing, but in rising every time we fall."

16. Accepting Accountability and Responsibility

A champion understands that when we refuse to accept accountability and responsibility for our performances, we relinquish control of those performances.

17. Willingness to Sacrifice

"Whatever it takes" attitude

18. Recognizing that we are a part of something bigger than our individual aspirations

A unified effort will always accomplish more than the collective efforts of a group of individuals.

19. Service

- Focus on our neighbor (teammates) will bring the best out of us.
- "Success is measured not by what you have gained for yourself but by what you have done for others."

20. "Team First" Attitude and Unconditional Support for the Team

- Support for the team even when I would prefer to do things differently
- Willingness to make personal sacrifices for the sake of the team (with a smile)
- Caring about my teammates and our team goals

21. Appreciating the Honor and Privilege

Of representing my country, city, sport, team, family, etc. and accepting the corresponding responsibility to do so with class and good sportsmanship (in both wins and losses).

22. Humility and Gratitude

Recognition that in addition to my own efforts, my success is due to the gifts of talent and opportunity, together with the support of others.

23. Integrity

Dictionary synonyms: uprightness, soundness of character, moral wholeness, trustworthiness (be a man/woman of your word)

24. Relentless Commitment to the Pursuit of Excellence

25. Strength of Character

Especially when put to the test.

26. Priorities, Principles, and Values

- Are consistent with your goals
- Are reflected in your thoughts, words, and actions

27. Understanding that true greatness is all about performing up to the best of my ability and striving to become the best that you can be (as an athlete and a person).

Dennis Pursley

During Dennis Pursley's coaching career, he was a five-time Olympic coach, a recipient of the US Olympic Committee Chair's Coaching Award, an American Swimming Coaches Association "Coach Of The Year," an American Swimming Coaches Association Hall of Fame inductee, and was recognized in 2003 as one of the "25 Most Influential People in the History of USA Swimming." He personally coached swimmers of both genders to world record performances and to the podium of the Olympic Games and/or the long course World Championships in all four competitive strokes and both individual medley events.

While a member of Plantation Swim Club and a student at Trinity High School in Louisville, Kentucky, Dennis was multiple times a state champion, team captain, and All American. After graduating in 1968, he attended the University of Alabama where he was an SEC champion, team captain, and earned undergraduate and graduate degrees in education. His coaching career began as a volunteer assistant coach under Coach Don Gambril at the University of Alabama while serving as the head coach of the University Aquatic Club. In 1974, Dennis returned to his hometown as the head coach of Louisville's Lakeside Swim Club. With Coach Pursley at the helm, Lakeside progressed from an unranked status with no regional or national qualifiers to a regional championship team title and a top 10 national championship finish. In 1979, he was appointed to the coaching staff of the USA Pan American Games team. In this competition, one of his swimmers, Mary T. Meagher, surprised the swimming world by establishing her first of several world records.

From Lakeside Swim Club, Coach Pursley moved on to assume the head coaching responsibilities for the Cincinnati Marlins and led them to three national championship team titles. Eleven swimmers on his 1980 championship team accounted for twenty-eight world rankings (top 25) in individual events, and eight Marlin relays were ranked among the top 25 in the world in that same year. After placing six swimmers on the 1980 USA Olympic Team who accounted for three world records (from Mary T Meagher and Bill Barrett) and four first-place world rankings, Coach Pursley was appointed to the USA Olympic Team coaching staff and was awarded 1980 "Coach of the Year" honors by the American Swimming Coaches Association.

In 1981, Coach Pursley was named the first head coach of the Australian Institute of Sport (AIS) where he served as the head coach of the combined team for two years and of the men's team until August, 1984. In the 1984 Olympic Games, the AIS led a resurgence in Australian swimming with a second place finish to the

United States in the medal count. Six of the AIS athletes who had trained under Pursley (four men and two women) accounted for half of Australia's medals. Only one of these athletes was ranked among the top 20 in the world (eighteenth) in 1983. After the 1984 Olympic Games, Coach Pursley began a three-year term as head coach for the Olympian Swim Club in Edmonton, Alberta, where his team progressed from fifth to first in provincial championship competition.

During the first decade of Coach Pursley's career, his swimmers accounted for seven world records, twelve American Records, and twenty US National Championship gold medals, as well as numerous medals in major international competitions, including the Olympic Games and the World Championships.

In 1989, Coach Pursley was appointed the first National Team Director of USA Swimming and was responsible for all aspects of the National Team program. During his fourteen-year tenure in this position, the medal production of the USA in international competition increased substantially. The USA team finished first in the medal count in both men's and women's competitions in all three Olympiads, culminating with thirty-three medals (fourteen gold) in the 2000 Olympics, which was described by "Sports Illustrated" magazine as the greatest team performance of all time. In recognition of his contributions, Coach Pursley was presented the United States Olympic Committee Chairman's Coaching Award for 2000.

Coach Pursley returned to the deck in 2003 as the head coach of the Brophy East Swim Team in Phoenix Arizona, and later that year, he was selected as one of the twenty-five most influential people in the history of USA Swimming. He was inducted into the American Swimming Coaches Hall of Fame in 2006. In 2008 he was named head coach of British Swimming and served in that capacity through the 2012 London Olympics.

After the 2012 Olympics, Coach Pursley returned to the University of Alabama as the head coach to lead his alma mater back to a position of national prominence in swimming and diving. Coach Pursley's second-year men's team was named "Breakout Team of the Year" by the College Swimming Coaches Association and went on to achieve six consecutive top 15 finishes in the NCAA Championships in his seven-year tenure, including four top 10 finishes. He was named University of Alabama men's "Coach of the Year" in 2016, and his team was named "University of Alabama Men's Team of the Year" in 2019. His women's team rewrote the school record books establishing new school records in seventeen of the nineteen events and finished in the scoring column in the NCAA Championships six consecutive years.

Dennis Pursley's life and career has been supported and inspired by his Catholic faith and his wife, Mary Jo, and five children, Brian, Lisa, David, Steven, and Joseph (JJ).